Why Do We Sleep

Facts about sleep, mechanisms and functions of sleep

Crown Loveth

Table of contents

Chapter 1

What is sleep ?

Before the dawn of contemporary sleep science in the early 1920s, sleep was thought of as a brain state that was not active. It was widely believed that as darkness fell, brain activity also decreased along with sensory inputs from the environment. In essence, scientists believed that while we sleep, the brain just shuts down and then wakes up and functions normally.

This theory was put to the test in 1929 when a device was developed that allowed scientists to record brain activity. Electroencephalograms (EEGs), which are recordings of brain activity, allowed scientists to see that sleep was a dynamic process during which the brain was occasionally quite active and was never completely asleep.

There are two basic forms of sleep, which were eventually identified through sleep research utilizing EEGs and other devices that recorded eye movements and muscle activity. Both the presence or absence of eye movements and typical electrical signals in the brain of a person who is asleep were used to identify these.

To sustain appropriate functioning and wellness, our bodies need to sleep. As a way of rejuvenating our bodies and brains, sleep is actually something we are hardwired to do every night. We leave our waking state and travel through a landscape of dreams and sleep for hours almost every night, and this is a tremendous transformation for almost everyone. Usually, when we wake up, we have very little to no memory of the previous few hours.

Everyone sleeps, yet most people struggle to describe what sleep actually is. All living things display a daily routine of activity and rest that is similar to the pattern of sleep and wakefulness that people experience every day. The following traits that go along with and in many ways characterize sleep have been identified by scientists by watching changes in behavior and responsiveness:

- During sleep, activity levels are low.
- In humans, lying down with our eyes closed is considered to be a common position for sleeping.

- In response to environmental stimuli, sleep reduces receptivity.
- It's quite simple to wake up from sleep (this distinguished sleep from other states of reduced consciousness, such as hibernation and coma).

Scientists have now characterized sleep in humans based on patterns of brain wave activity and other physiological changes as a result of studies of behavioral changes that occur during sleep and concurrent physical changes. As a result, the definition of sleep is defined as a state marked by changes in breathing, heart rate, body temperature, and other physiological activities. Now, sleep may be separated from awake by a reduced capacity to respond to stimuli, but it is still more responsive than a coma or disorders of consciousness, with sleep revealing distinct, active brain patterns.

How does sleep work?

In addition to being a spontaneous activity, sleep also exhibits dynamic characteristics as seen by how it interacts with the surrounding environment. During sleep, the perception of external stimuli is diminished but not completely eliminated. Even the exact brain reactions to stimulus from outside sources when you are sleeping have been demonstrated by functional brain imaging.

There are two essentially different forms of sleep: rapid eye movement (REM) sleep, which is linked to active dreaming, and non-rapid eye movement (NREM) sleep.

Physiologists classify REM and non-REM sleep as separate behavioral states because of their striking differences. Deep sleep, also known as slow-wave sleep, follows non-REM sleep and takes place after a transitional phase. Body temperature and pulse rate drop during this stage, while brain energy consumption decreases. The fraction of sleep time that is spent in REM sleep, sometimes referred to as paradoxical sleep, is less. It is the primary trigger for dreams (or nightmares) and is accompanied by jerky eye movements, rapid and disorganized brain waves, loss of muscular tone, and suspension of homeostasis.

NREM is broken down into three stages by the American Academy of Sleep Medicine (AASM): N1, N2, and N3. N3 is also known as delta sleep or slow-wave sleep. Normal progression throughout the entire time is N1 -> N2 -> N3 -> N2 -> REM. REM sleep happens when a person transitions from a deep sleep to stage 2 or 1. While the fraction of REM sleep increases in the two cycles right before natural waking, deep sleep (stage N3) is more prevalent earlier in the night.

Skeletal muscle activity typically shows a gradual decrease in amplitude when a person moves from being awake to N1, N2, and N3 sleep. The lowest skeletal muscle tone is related to REM sleep. The sleep cycle is cyclical over a typical night, with the start of sleep being followed by a quick decline to deep stage N3 sleep within the first hour. Following this, NREM and REM sleep alternate in cycles every 60 to 90 minutes for the remainder of the night. Most N3 sleep typically takes place in the early part of the night, whereas most REM sleep happens in the second half. It is yet unknown how fully biological and clinically significant this "ultradian" cycle of sleep depth is.

In summary, sleep is an actively controlled process that is heavily influenced by circadian effects entrained to the 24-hour day and by homeostatic impacts that collect throughout continued awake and dissipate during sleep. A well-defined subcortical network of brain areas controls the transitions between sleep and wakefulness, and sleep has a distinctive underlying architecture characterized by a regular alternation between NREM and REM stages. Different hormonal rhythms that exert potential major impacts on metabolism and glucose homeostasis are also present throughout sleep and wakefulness.

Chapter 2

What are the stages of sleep?

Rapid eye movement (REM) sleep and non-rapid eye movement (NREM) sleep are the two major categories of sleep phases. NREM is further broken down into the phases N1, N2, and N3. N1 – N2 – N3 – N2 – REM is the typical progression of the whole sleep cycle. Therefore, there are four phases of sleep: one for rapid eye movement (REM) sleep and three for non-REM (NREM). These stages are based on an investigation of brain activity during sleep, which reveals distinctive patterns that distinguish each stage.

Sleep stages	Type of sleep	Other names	Normal length
Stage 1	NREM	N1	1-5 minutes
Stage 2	NREM	N2	10-60 minutes
Stage 3	NREM	N3, slow wave sleep, delta sleep, deep sleep	20-40 minutes
Stage 4	REM	REM sleep	10-60 minutes

Sleep architecture is the term used to describe how a person's sleep is broken down into numerous cycles and phases. In a hypnogram, the visual representation of this sleep architecture may be seen if someone has a sleep study.

NREM Sleep Patterns

There are three distinct phases of NREM sleep. It becomes more difficult to awaken someone from sleep the deeper their stage of NREM sleep is.

Stage 1 / N1

Stage 1 often lasts between one and five minutes and is referred to as the "dozing off" stage.

Although the body hasn't completely relaxed during N1 sleep, the functions of the body and brain start to slow down with brief intervals of movement (twitches). During this period of sleep, there are slight changes in brain activity. Although it's simple to wake someone up during this stage of sleep, if they aren't bothered, they can easily transition into stage 2 of sleep. An uninterrupted sleeper may not spend much more time in stage 1 as the night goes on as they cycle through subsequent sleep cycles. Stage 1 of the EEG shows a change from alertness, which is characterized by repetitive alpha waves, to low-voltage, mixed-frequency waves. The frequency of alpha waves, which are connected to a wakeful state of relaxation, ranges from 8 to 13 cycles per second.

Stage 2 / N2

Stage 2 of the process sees the body go into a more passive state with lowered body temperature, relaxed muscles, and slower breathing and heart rate. Eye movement pauses and brain waves display a new pattern simultaneously. Overall, brain activity decreases during stage 2 sleep, but there are brief bursts of activity that actually work to prevent being awakened by outside stimuli. As a result, stage 2 sleepers need stronger external stimulation to awaken than those in stage 1 sleep. During the initial sleep cycle, stage 2 sleep might continue for 10 to 25 minutes, and each subsequent N2 stage can get longer as the night goes on. Generally speaking, N2 sleep accounts for around half of a person's total sleep time. Around 45 to 55 percent of the entire sleep experience occurs in stage 2. The existence of sleep spindles and K-complexes on an EEG is indicative of relatively low-voltage, mixed-frequency activity in the brain. Sleep spindles are thought to be crucial for the formation of new memories. People who master a new skill have a sleep spindle density that is noticeably higher than people in a control group.

Stage 3 / N3

It is more difficult to rouse someone up if they are in stage three sleep, commonly known as deep slumber. As the body continues to relax, N3 sleep results in a reduction in muscle tone, pulse, and breathing rate. Delta waves, a recognized pattern of brain activity, are present at this time. Because of this, stage 3 is also known as delta sleep or slow-wave sleep (SWS). This phase, according to experts, is essential to restorative sleep because it enables physical healing and growth. It could also strengthen the immune system and other vital body functions. Although brain activity is decreased, there is evidence that deep sleep improves memory, creativity, and perceptive thinking. The first half of the night is when we are sleeping deeply the most. N3 phases frequently last 20 to 40 minutes during the early sleep cycles. These phases of sleep become shorter as you sleep longer and more time is spent in REM sleep. It makes up around 15 to 20 percent of sleep. An increase in high-voltage, slow-wave activity is visible in the EEG.

REM Sleep Patterns

The amount of brain activity increases during REM sleep and approaches levels seen while awake. The muscles in the body temporarily paralyze at the same moment, with the exception of the muscles that govern respiration and the eyes. The term for this stage comes from the fact that while the eyelids are closed, they may be seen moving fast. It is thought that REM sleep is crucial for cognitive processes including memory, learning, and creativity. The intense increase in brain activity during REM sleep explains why those who have vivid dreams report having them more frequently. Though dreams can happen at any stage of sleep, they are less frequent and strong during the NREM cycles. In a typical sleep cycle, you don't reach a REM sleep state until after roughly 90 minutes of sleep.

The length of REM periods increases during the night, especially in the second half. Early REM stages may only last a few minutes, while later stages might endure for almost an hour. Around 25% of adult sleep is made up of REM phases overall. Age, the amount of recent sleep or wakefulness, the time of day or night relative to an individual's internal clock, other behaviors prior to sleep such as exercise, stress, environmental conditions such as temperature and light, and various chemicals are just a few of the variables that can affect sleep patterns. For instance, during the first year of life, REM sleep frequently starts before NREM sleep.

Despite being substantially shorter than the 90-minute cycles that occur in adults, the cyclical alternation of NREM-REM sleep is present in babies from birth and lasts for 50 to 60 minutes. After two to six months, nocturnal sleep is entirely consolidated, and the NREM sleep phases EEG patterns are fully formed. Even while the amount of slow-wave sleep does not alter with time, it is highest in young children and slowly declines with age. The structure and operation of the brain may have changed as a result of this. By the time newborns are two years old, their brains are 90% the size of an adult's brain, with the majority of this brain development taking place during the stage of life with the highest rate of sleep. Children's capacity to accomplish cognitive activities is influenced by how much time they spend sleeping. Children who sleep through the night and experience minimal nighttime awakenings are more likely to have easy temperaments and greater cognitive abilities than other kids.

Chapter 3

What are the sleep mechanisms?

Most physiological processes in complex organisms are regulated by two systems. There is the idea of homeostasis, where physiological variables are controlled to stay relatively constant across time and close to a predetermined value. Contrarily, the idea of circadian regulation alters the level of each variable for optimal performance at the appropriate time of day. Mrosovsky(1990) created the word "Rheostasis" to combine the two.

Homeostasis and the circadian rhythm, two internal biological processes, collaborate to control when you are awake and asleep.

Circadian rhythms control a vast range of bodily processes, including hormone release, body temperature regulation, and daily variations in wakefulness. They dictate when you go to sleep, make you drowsy at night, and make you more likely to wake up in the morning without an alarm. The majority of circadian rhythms are managed by your body's biological clock, which is based on an approximately 24-hour day. Environmental signals (such as light and temperature) that indicate the actual time of day help synchronize circadian rhythms, but they don't need to be present for them to function.

Therefore, the suprachiasmatic nucleus (or nuclei) (SCN), a pair of separate groupings of cells in the hypothalamus, houses the main circadian clock in mammals. The complete lack of a consistent sleep-wake cycle is caused by the destruction of the SCN. It is via the eyes that the SCN learns about light. Traditional vision is made possible by the presence of "classical" photoreceptors in the retina of the eye (referred to as "rods" and "cones"). But in addition, the retina has specialized ganglion cells that project directly to the SCN and are photosensitive, aiding in the synchronization of the body's main circadian clock. The retinohypothalamic tract is a conduit that carries information from these cells to the SCN, which is where the photopigment melanopsin is found. When SCN cells are taken out and cultured, they continue to retain their own rhythm even in the absence of environmental signals. The SCN processes the information about day and night lengths received from the retina and sends it to the pineal gland, a small organ situated on the epithalamus and resembling a pine cone. The pineal gland releases the hormone melatonin in response. Melatonin secretion rises at night and declines throughout the day, and its presence tells us how long the night is. Numerous investigations have shown that pineal melatonin modulates circadian rhythms of activity and other activities by feeding back on SCN rhythmicity.

The classic phase markers for measuring the timing of a mammal's circadian rhythm are:

1. Melatonin secretion by the pineal gland,

2. Core body temperature minimum, and

3. Plasma level of cortisol

The regulation of sleep enables organisms to make up for lost sleep (caused, for example, by sleep deprivation) or excess sleep (e.g by prolonging sleep in the morning or by napping).

Your sleep needs are monitored by sleep-wake homeostasis. The body is reminded to go to bed at a set time, and the homeostatic sleep drive controls how deep the sleep is. Every hour you spend awake, this sleep urge grows stronger, and after a period of sleep deprivation, it drives you to sleep longer and deeper. The equilibrium between waking and sleeping is controlled by sleep homeostasis. Departures from a normal reference sleep level are resisted by homeostatic processes. The homeostatic process, A Process S, grows as an exponential saturating function when awake and shrinks as an exponential function while sleeping. Slow-wave activity during non-REM sleep is a sign that Process S is waning. A homeostatic mechanism, the circadian system, and their interactions control the daily monophasic or biphasic sleep-wake cycle, which is common for humans, as well as the polyphasic sleep-wake cycles in animals. Sleep length and sleep intensity, to a lesser extent, are the two key controlled factors (or the amount of sleep). While the circadian clock controls sleep timing, the homeostatic system controls the amount of sleep.

Along with other variables, human developmental phases and maturation have an impact on the homeostasis of sleep (diet, mental health e.t.c.). Prepubescent or early pubescent children see a higher rise in homeostatic sleep pressure during waking than mature adolescents, whereas both developmental groups experience a similar decline in Process S. These age-related variations suggest that the young brain generates slow waves with less time awake than the adult brain. Some could argue that the change in circadian phase markers between developing groups and the differences in scheduled bedtime between baseline and recovery sleep affected the calculation of homeostatic parameters. However, it was found that sleep homeostasis is essentially independent of the circadian timing system.

Thus, both the homeostatic and circadian mechanisms control sleep. The majority of sleep-related factors, including sleepiness and alertness, are governed by these two processes when they work together. It is well recognized that the two processes can each function independently, but they can also both have an additive or more complicated effect on factors connected to sleep and sleep cycles. It is evident that the circadian clock has a significant influence on sleep schedule, particularly in humans. Additionally, sleep homeostatic processes have a significant role in the depth and maintenance of sleep. Incorporating the two regulatory processes was proposed in the "two process" model of sleep regulation.

The fundamental characteristics of sleep regulation, according to this theory, are determined by the interaction of a homeostatic process (process S), which depends on how much time was spent awake and sleeping in the past, and a process (process C) governed by the circadian pacemaker. Since the model's concepts are straightforward to apply to a wide range of sleep research problems, it has become the most widely used model in the area of sleep during the past 30 years and has sparked a significant amount of new research. This is the fundamental justification for using it here as a foundation to explore the evidence of a purported reciprocal connection between the two processes. In the two-process concept, Process S stands for sleep homeostasis or sleep debt, which rises when awake and falls asleep within a range that oscillates with a regularity that is entrained to day and night by the circadian pacemaker. S causes awakening when it approaches the lower threshold, and sleep when it hits the upper threshold. The most significant interactions between the two processes take place when S crosses either the higher threshold, transitioning from waking to sleep, or the lower threshold, transitioning from sleep to waking. One would wonder whether this is the only time during the day that the two speak and collaborate. It is understood that the two processes are capable of operating apart from one another.

Chapter 4

Why do we need sleep?

In this chapter we will be considering the major functions of sleep clarifying the reasons why we need good and quality sleep. Sleep plays an essential role in many vital physiologic functions including development, energy conservation, brain waste clearance, and modulation of immune responses, cognition, performance, disease, vigilance, and psychological conditions.

Sleep function in physical restoration

Due to the fact that sleep is thought to be important for energy conservation and that it is known that sleeping less leads to higher daily energy expenditure, sleep is thought to be necessary. Given that sleep has a lower metabolic rate than wakefulness, it's possible that biological functions can be carried out during sleep at a lower total energy cost. The observation that hormones released during sleep, such as growth hormone, have a predominant anabolic function, as opposed to hormones associated with wakefulness, which tend to have a catabolic effect, is a major argument in favor of the restorative function of sleep. Cortisol, for example, is suppressed during sleep and the amplitude of the circadian cortisol decline is dampened by sleep restriction.

Growth hormone levels significantly decrease during sleep deprivation. The majority of growth hormone pulses happen during slow-wave sleep (SWS), with the majority of pulses happening immediately after sleep onset in the first period of SWS sleep. Since sleep is related with reduced energy expenditure and sleep deprivation with higher total daily energy expenditure, sleep is thought to be important for energy conservation. Given that sleep has a lower metabolic rate than wakefulness, it's possible that biological activities taking place while we sleep use less energy overall.

Sleep function in energy conservation

The hypothesis that sleep serves the purpose of energy conservation is supported by the fact that a decrease in body temperature of 1 to 2 degrees celsius during sleep can cause humans to use up to 10% less energy. This temperature reduction during sleep is especially significant when there is little to gain from being awake and active. Both a decrease in body and brain activity when you sleep and a drop of the body's temperature regulation set point are sources of the energy savings. The significant energy savings are caused by the lowering of the set point while you sleep. According to the energy conservation hypothesis, the primary purpose of sleep is to lower a person's energy needs during the hours of the day and night when it is least effective to go food hunting.

The dynamic state-dependent metabolic partitioning and resource optimization proposed by recent energy allocation theory sees sleep-wake cycle as a behavioral approach encouraging energy saving. The partitioning of metabolic activities by behavioral state happens at the level of the entire organism and is not limited to a particular organ or structure, which is a fundamental tenet of this theory. Thus, resource optimization through sleep-wake cycle boosts overall energy savings beyond what a single organ system might otherwise accomplish.

Sleep function in learning and memory

For the rest of the body, such as the muscles, passive rest may be helpful, but the brain does not benefit from rest in the same way. The only thing that will work is sleep. The brain is still quite busy even while you are relaxing quietly, practicing meditation, or "zoning out." When brain activity is decreased, biological advantages can be obtained more quickly. This criterion can only be satisfied during N3, the slow wave sleep stage.This activity reduction applies to the cerebrum but not to the brainstem. The brainstem's functions are fixedly programmed, with limited room for adaptation or modification. The cerebrum, in contrast, is malleable, allowing for greater behavioral and learning flexibility but needing more care and maintenance.

As a result, if sleep has any purpose at all, it is probably to help the higher portions of the brain by reducing their level of activity. As a result of nocturnal sleep and daytime naps, memory processes have been demonstrated to be stabilized, strengthened (accelerated and/or integrated), and memories are more consolidated. Although this is task-specific, it has been shown that some sleep phases can enhance a person's memory. Slow-wave sleep is generally thought to improve declarative memories, but rapid eye movement (REM) sleep is thought to improve non-declarative memories. Sleep is necessary for memory processing, including reactivation, analysis, alteration, and consolidation or reconsolidation of short-term memory. The memory representation is transformed and qualitatively reorganized as a result of the active system consolidation process, which is thought to occur while we sleep. The "gist" is taken from the newly encoded memory material and incorporated into the long-term knowledge networks. Accordingly, sleep favors memory consolidation processes that are incompatible with the effective encoding and retrieval of stimuli, as required while coping with environmental demands in the wake phase. Sleep and wakefulness thus appear to be associated with different and mutually exclusive modes of memory processing.

Sleep function in behavioral and emotional adaptation

It is clear that one function of sleep is mood regulation because sleep loss tends to raise negative mood and decrease happy mood in most persons. Numerous research have demonstrated that recent sleep quantity and quality have an impact on non-depressed people's morning mood. A good night's rest enhances mood in the morning. One night of sleep deprivation results in considerably poorer morning mood scores for these individuals. In general, sleep improves mood. It has been demonstrated that sleep deprivation decreases the positive gain that results from pleasant or goal-directed activities while increasing the negative emotional effects of disruptive waking occurrences. Additionally, it has been shown that sleep has a significant impact on how conditioned fear is modulated. If the conditioned stimulus (the tone) is offered in an environment that is either risky or safe, sleep preferentially changes the appropriate expression of fear relative to time spent awake.

Therefore, those who sleep exhibit considerably more adaptable forms of fear, either maintaining or reducing fear responses depending on whether there are safe or risky contextual cues present. Therefore, based on environmental information signaling threat or safety, sleep enables the most suitable or "intelligent" expression of conditioned fear. Overall, the results of trials on fear conditioning show that REM sleep, as well as other types of sleep, supports adaptive fear responses on a variety of levels. The advantages of these processes support the appropriate production and maintenance of fear responses in risky situations while limiting fear responses to non-threatening situations. The same processes, however, are hampered by sleep deprivation in part because the prefrontal cortex's top-down control over limbic areas in the subcortical brain is lost. This is especially important in a clinical setting because fear-related disorders like specific phobia and post-traumatic stress disorder (PTSD), the latter of which is associated with significant sleep disruption, are characterized by deficits in the extinction of fear and in the capacity to use context-relevant information appropriately.

Functions of the sleep stages

NREM

N3 is essential for body restoration. Your subsequent N3 becomes more severe the longer you are awake. On the other hand, N3 intensity falls off rapidly the longer you sleep. One theory is that the longer you remain awake, the more your body will deteriorate and/or use up resources that can only be replenished during N3. An rise in anabolic hormones and a reduction in catabolic hormones are observed in the body during NREMS. While catabolic hormones tend to exhaust the body, anabolic hormones tend to build up and repair the body. In mature humans, growth hormone is only present during the first N3 phase of the night. For children, N3 is when it is even more common. During NREMS, the immune system's capabilities grow. Additionally, it has been demonstrated that getting extra sleep as a result of increased sleepiness brought on by a number of ailments helps patients recover from their illnesses. Evidence from recent studies suggests that N2 may be crucial for the ongoing execution of procedural memory tasks, such as simple motor skill tests.

REM

It has been noted that while some of REM sleep capabilities appear to be preparatory, others are adaptive. To put it another way, whereas certain functions prepare an organism for potential future requirements by anticipating them, others react to past experiences by making an effort to make the most of them. The brain's stimulation for healthy growth, its repair and maintenance, and the exercise of brain circuits for genetically based behaviors are some of the preparatory activities.

These processes aid in ensuring that the brain is prepared to react correctly when needed in the future. The adaptive functions also include the psychological advantages of dreams, mood regulation, and memory work on new learning. Because REM sleep is good for growth, it lasts longer when a fetus or a newborn is developing. Adults' REM sleep is less intense than it was previously, but it still exists. The functional channels of intercellular communication between brain cells are maintained and self-correct through this predictable internal source of stimulus. It has been proposed that REM sleep helps maintain not just the motor and sensory systems but also the brain circuits responsible for inherited inherent behaviors. REM sleep is beneficial for brain restoration throughout life because certain neurotransmitters, such as catecholamines and hypocretin, which are heavily used when awake, may need to have their levels replenished, their receptors restored, or other related mechanisms are revitalized during REM sleep when the cells that use them are much less active. The purpose of REM sleep is to keep the brain warm as you sleep, especially the brainstem, as much of your body cools. The expression of drives may be influenced by REM sleep, according to a theory.

The animal's capacity to satisfy its waking drive is modulated to provide it more adaptability and flexibility. Because the settings for memory consolidation may be ideal during REM sleep, REM sleep is believed to be vital for memory. The brain is free from competing functions during REM sleep, there is a high rate of protein synthesis compatible with preservation of memory-related neuronal components, and the information flow during REM sleep reverses, flowing from the neocortex to the hippocampus instead. The modulation of mood and emotions is thought to depend significantly on REM sleep. Most people are believed to be more adaptable and flexible when awake as a result of REM sleep since it is associated with "improved successful adjustment" and "better interpersonal competence and creativity."

However, it appears that sleep benefits the brain more than the rest of the body overall. The worst effects of lack of regular sleep are seen in mental functioning. There is growing evidence that this happens because sleep is necessary for regular brain function, particularly for preserving neuronal architecture and brain chemistry within specified bounds while simultaneously allowing for plasticity required for memory consolidation. For this maintenance to take place without being impeded by sensory inputs and motor outputs, unconsciousness during sleep may be a need. In other words, to carry out necessary maintenance, the brain must be virtually "off line." Simple relaxed wakefulness does not suffice.

Chapter 5

What are sleep parameters?

Sleep parameters are useful in assessing our quality of sleep and identifying our unique sleeping patterns. When conducting a sleep study, they are often taken into account. The typical sleep parameters are as follows: **Sleep latency (SL)** is the interval between turning out the lights and the first epoch of any sleep stage. **Total sleep time (TST)** is the amount of time in minutes that a person spends sleeping throughout a sleeping session. **REM latency**, the amount of time it takes a person to enter their first REM sleep state following the darkness; the period in minutes that a person is awake following the onset of sleep, counting from that point until they are completely awake and do not try to fall back asleep; **Number of awakenings (NA),** the number of times a person transitions from sleep to waking, and **sleep efficiency (SE),** the proportion of total time in bed that is actually spent sleeping.

Total sleep time (TST)

The total quantity of sleep time is the sum of all sleep hours recorded over the whole recording period. This covers the period from the start of sleep to the end of sleep, and it is divided into minutes for Stage N1 sleep, Stage N2 sleep, Stage N3 sleep, and rapid eye movement (REM) sleep. Minutes are used to describe all of these times. A little amount of total sleep time may be a sign that the patient slept for a shorter amount of time than necessary owing to non-medical or physiological causes, certain medical conditions or sleep disorders, or as a side effect of medication.Long periods of complete sleep might be a sign of previous sleep deprivation, certain illnesses, or drug side effects. Even when there is an apparent normal total amount of sleep time, severe sleep fragmentation, as characterized by frequent awakenings and/or stage transitions, can lead to complaints of non-restorative sleep. Stage N1 sleep accounts for around 5% of all adult sleep time, Stage N2 for 50%, and Stage N3 for 20%. The final 25% of sleep is in the REM period.

Sleep latency (SL)

The amount of time between turning out the lights and the first sleep stage's initial epoch is known as sleep latency (including stage N1). The sleep delay is recorded as 20 minutes if no signs of sleep are present. It is the period of time it takes you to go from a fully aware state to sleep. Each individual has a different sleep delay. You can tell how much and what kind of sleep you're receiving by looking at your sleep latency and how soon you enter rapid eye movement (REM) sleep. One of the most crucial variables in a sleep research is likely sleep latency.

Sleep latency is defined as the amount of time between the time the lights are turned out (lights out) and the time the person actually falls asleep, as seen by changes in their EEG and other behavioral characteristics during sleep. The duration of sleep is measured by the number of minutes it takes from the moment the lights go off to the first epoch that is recorded as sleep. Sleep latency also shows if the person's sleep diary was read with appropriate care and whether the patient's scheduled bedtime at home was within a few hours of the lights-out time. Obviously, sleep latency would be spuriously long if the lights were put out before the person usually goes to bed, and the person might not start to nod off until his or her typical bedtime is reached. Similar to this, if the patient goes to bed later than normal, there will be sleepiness and an artificially short sleep latency will be recorded. It is crucial that the individual's typical sleep pattern and estimated "lights out" time be taken into account while designing their sleep research.

Rapid eye movement latency (REM Latency)

Also referred to as REM latency, rapid eye movement latency. The duration between the start of sleep and the first REM sleep epoch is known as rapid eye movement latency, and it is dependent on each person's sleep latency. Every 90 to 120 minutes throughout the course of the night, REM sleep cycles occur. A variety of sleep disorders are thought to have variations in REM sleep latency as possible biological indicators. Medication side effects, sleep deprivation, and irregular circadian rhythms all have a strong impact on REM sleep. Therefore, it is crucial to assess the patients' current medicines as well as the quality of their sleep the night before the sleep study. Withdrawal from monoamine oxidase inhibitors (MAOIs) or tricyclic antidepressants (TCAs) may cause a short REM latency period. Alcohol withdrawal, barbiturate withdrawal, and amphetamine withdrawal can all reduce the REM latency time. Short REM latency may also be seen in those with narcolepsy, sleep apnea, and depressive histories. Similar to how REM-suppressing drugs like TCAs, MAOIs, amphetamine, barbiturates, and alcohol may cause extended REM latency. Long REM sleep latency can also be caused by sleep apnea and intermittent limb movement during sleep.

Wake after sleep onset (WASO)

WASO, sometimes referred to as wake after sleep onset This is used to describe intervals of awake that follow a clear sleep start. The alertness measured by this characteristic does not include the wakefulness just before falling asleep. Sleep fragmentation is better reflected by WASO time. In sleep research, the statistic known as Wake Moment After Sleep Onset (WASO) is used to calculate how long an individual is awake between the time they initially fall asleep and the point at which they are completely alert and do not try to fall back asleep. This statistic often uses minutes as its unit of measurement. When sleep studies are done on persons who have trouble falling asleep, the wake time after sleep onset (WASO) is assessed.

The inability to fall asleep is more common in those who have sleep apnea, stress, insomnia, RLS, weak bladders, or arthritis. Sleep problems are also often experienced by pregnant or menopausal women. One of the variables used to calculate the length of the sleep period in sleep studies is the wake time after the start of sleep. Sleep Period Time is calculated as the total of total sleep time and wake time following the commencement of sleep. Overheating while sleeping, noise disturbances, the need to use the restroom in the middle of the night, or even underlying medical disorders like sleep apnea and insomnia, are just a few of the factors that can contribute to WASO. A person's ability to sleep through the night may also be impacted by their ability to manage worry or stressful life events.

Sleep efficiency

The percentage of a person's total time in bed that is actually spent sleeping is known as sleep efficiency. The sum of stages N1, N2, N3, and REM sleep is computed, then that number is multiplied by 100 and divided by the entire amount of time spent in bed. The patient's overall level of sleep efficiency can be determined, but it does not differentiate between several, brief wakeful episodes. Extended sleep latency and long sleep offset to light on time, with otherwise normal quantity and quality of sleep in between, may cause a poor sleep efficiency. Numerous laboratories record total wake time, which is the duration of wakefulness over the whole recording period in minutes following the start of sleep.

The total quantity provides a broad evaluation of the overall sleep quality. Total sleep time is equal to total wake time. A low total wake time percent and a high total sleep time percent are always related. A sleep efficiency of 80% or above is regarded as normal. To reach an 80% or better level of sleep efficiency, for instance, a person needs to spend at least 6.4 hours or more sleeping if they spend 8 hours in bed (from 10 p.m. to 6 a.m.). The majority of young, healthy persons have sleep efficiency levels exceeding 90%. Other studies have also suggested that the denominator in the SE equation should not be TIB, but rather the time period that starts with the first attempt to sleep and ends when the person finally wakes and no longer attempts to sleep. There have been disagreements regarding the measurement of sleep efficiency in relation to the commonly used formula, which is commonly defined as the ratio of total sleep time (TST) to time in bed (TIB).

Number of awakenings

The phrase "number of awakenings" describes how frequently someone switches between being asleep and waking. There were no statistically significant variations between the genders in the average number of awakenings, according to a National Institutes of Health research. They did discover that elderly people typically woke up more often, though. Actually, six times a night is about how often people awaken on average. includes any instances of waking while a person is in bed (TIB). The number of times the person was awake while in bed (for one minute or more) is what is being counted (TIB). Adults often awaken 2 to 6 times per night, which is considered to be a normal number. Sometimes the time in bed (TIB) is used to describe this sleep parameter instead of the sleep onset to sleep offset interval, which will indicate the number of awakenings between sleep onset and sleep offset.

Chapter 6

Conclusion

Sleep is a daily occurrence in our everyday lives, while we may not understand why it is so important even though everyone deems it a necessity since the body requires it and we can not always fight the body's need. Just like eating healthy is important to enjoying a good and productive life so likewise sleep is also important for our healthy wellbeing and sleep deprivation can lead to a lot of medical complications. Therefore the importance of a short read like this to educate us on the mechanics of sleep and how it affects our body and health.

www.ingramcontent.com/pod-product-compliance
Lightning Source LLC
Chambersburg PA
CBHW051701250726
48653CB00007B/2789